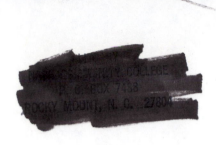

W9-CBU-227

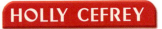
HOLLY CEFREY

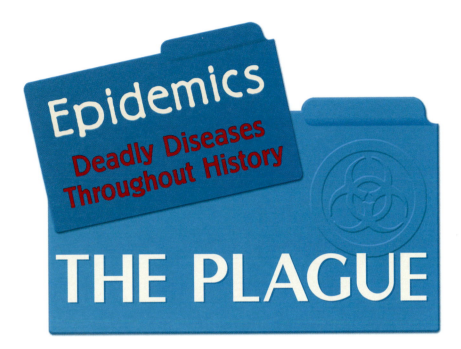
Epidemics
Deadly Diseases
Throughout History

THE PLAGUE

The Rosen Publishing Group, Inc.
New York

To Richard, Ethan, Elaine, and Dean

Published in 2001 by The Rosen Publishing Group, Inc.
29 East 21st Street, New York, NY 10010

First Edition

Library of Congress Cataloging-in-Publication Data

Cefrey, Holly.
The plague / by Holly Cefrey. — 1st ed.
    p. cm. — (Epidemics)
Includes bibliographical references and index.
ISBN 0-8239-3343-1
1. Plague—Juvenile literature. [1. Plague. 2. Diseases.] I.
Epidemics!
RC171 .C44 2001
614.5′732--dc21

00-010786

Cover image: A gram stain of *Yersinia pestis*, the bacterium that causes the bubonic plague.

Manufactured in the United States of America

CONTENTS

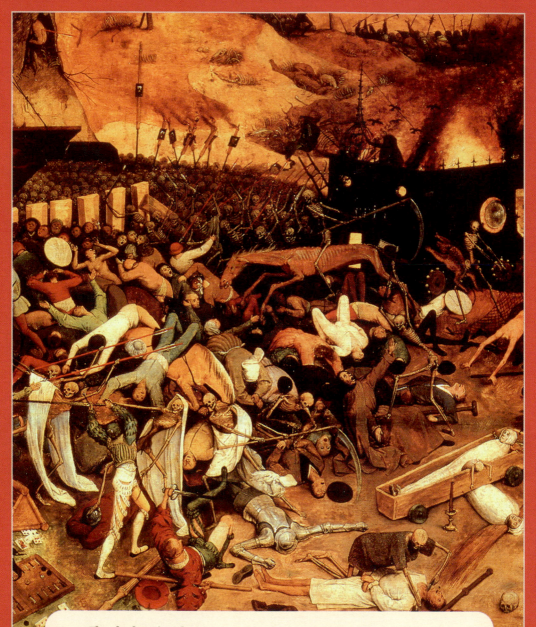

The bubonic plague, or Black Death, devastated Europe and Asia during the fourteenth century.

INTRODUCTION

I was born in Genoa, which was one of the major trading ports of the West. From our city all of Europe could have access to the finest silks and goods from places as far away as China. My father, a merchant, was one of the many people who made trips along the trade routes to bring goods to our part of the world. He traveled by ship to other trading ports and by caravan along the Silk Road. My father would take gold, precious metals, and fabrics from our area to trade for furs, ceramics, bronze weapons, and spices from other areas. Our people, the Genoese, had established trading posts all along the major trading routes. Sometimes my father was sent to stay at these posts for months at a time. When he would return from a trip, my mother, sister, and I would run to greet him at the shore. We were always excited to see him and amazed by the interesting things he would bring back with him.

One day we rushed to the port to welcome Father home. He had been gone for nearly three months, and we were very excited to see him. When we arrived at the dock, however, we were saddened to find that his ship had arrived without him. Many of the men on board looked very ill. One sailor, a friend of our father, took Mother aside and whispered something to her. She became very frightened. As the sailor walked away, we tugged at Mother's dress, asking her where Father was. She said that something was wrong and quickly escorted us back into town.

When we arrived at home, Mother sat us down and told us about a plague that had been killing people in countries far to the east of Genoa. Mother explained that a plague is a serious, contagious disease. People who got the plague became so sick that priests and doctors could not help them. Then Mother told us the most shocking news of all: Father had caught the plague and had died long before his ship had sailed home.

Before that fateful day, we had always believed that people who became sick were being punished by God for committing sins. Our parents always asked us to pray for anyone who had developed sickness. Now we were not so sure. Mother had heard that this plague was so dangerous that people could get sick by merely being in the same room with a sick person.

Within weeks, many people in my city were ill and dying. Mother had sent word to her sister in Paris that she would be sending my sister and me to Paris until the sickness passed. On the day that we left, our neighbor died. She died alone in her bed. Her husband and children had left her when she became ill, as they were scared to catch her sickness. The plague scared people so much that more and more families became separated. It was hard for us to leave Mother, but she insisted that we go. She asked me to be brave and to look after my sister.

A few months after my sister and I arrived in Paris, the plague struck there, too. This time, I stayed to witness its terrible devastation. My

AD 541–544

Justinian's plague ravages northern Africa, western Asia, and southern Europe.

1334

The Black Plague occurs in Asia.

1335–1345

The Black Plague is carried west along the Silk Road into western Asia and the Middle East.

1347

The Black Plague strikes the Italian peninsula.

sister soon became ill. It started with a head-ache and chills, and soon she had growths the size of eggs under the skin on her legs. My sister passed away within three days of getting the plague. My cousins fell victim to the plague as well. I feared that the plague would continue to ravage the city until no one was left.

—Diary entry of an unknown child, July 1348

The plague that struck Asia and Europe during the fourteenth century is known as the Black Plague or the Black Death. The Black Plague is one of the most important and devastating events in

1348
The plague spreads to France, England, Ireland, and Germany.

1349
The Black Plague is carried to Norway and Scotland.

1351
The plague strikes Russia.

1352
The plague forms a deadly ring around Europe.

(continued)

European and Asian history. The Black Plague killed huge numbers of people. Some areas of Europe were so devastated that there were not enough people left to bury the dead. Asia was hit hard as well. About two-thirds of the people of China were killed by the plague.

Medieval Medicine

Before the Black Plague struck, people held various beliefs as to why illness occurred. Most people's beliefs about illness were based on myths and superstitions. Some people believed that bad vapors, or clouds of gas, were the cause of illness. It

1893
An outbreak of the plague in China starts the modern pandemic.

1894
Alexandre Yersin discovers the organism that causes the bubonic plague.

1896
The first plague vaccine is invented by Waldemar Haffkine.

was also believed that illness developed as a form of divine wrath, or punishment from God. People thought that they were being punished because of sins or bad deeds.

Medieval doctors, following the teachings of the ancient Greeks and Romans, believed that illness was due to an imbalance of the humors, or fluids, in the human body. They believed that there were four fluids in the body: blood, phlegm, black bile, and yellow bile. Bodily functions, such as sweating, crying, or having bowel movements were thought to keep the humors in balance by releasing extra fluids. It was thought that as long as the fluids stayed in balance, a person would be healthy.

When a person became ill, it was believed that his or her humors were out of balance. Medieval doctors thought that the humors became unbalanced when one or more of the fluids were not released properly by the body. Extra amounts of fluid were believed to be the cause of health and personality problems. Because a person's illness was thought to be caused by his or her own fluid imbalance, doctors treated each case of illness uniquely. The fact that many diseases are caused by germs, bacteria, and viruses had not been discovered yet.

Bloodletting and Cupping

In the fourteenth century, medicine was still a primitive practice. Most medical treatments were based on the idea that the body contained excess fluids that needed to be released. Many of these treatments were quite painful, and in most cases did the patient more harm than good. One popular treatment, called bloodletting, was often performed in order to balance the fluids of an ill patient. The patient was cut and allowed to bleed into a bowl. Blood was drained until the patient felt faint. In some cases, bloodletting was done through the use of blood-sucking leeches.

Another common treatment was called cupping. Doctors heated cups and placed them on the skin of the infected patient. As the cups cooled, suction was

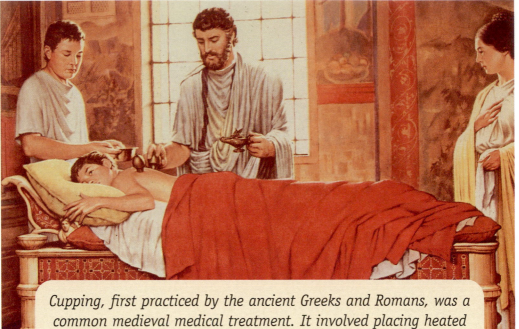

Cupping, first practiced by the ancient Greeks and Romans, was a common medieval medical treatment. It involved placing heated cups on the skin of an infected patient in order to draw out excess fluid that was believed to be the cause of illness.

created. The suction of the cooling cups caused the skin under the cup to become swollen. The swollen areas of skin were believed to be filled with excess body fluids. By bringing the extra fluids to the surface, health was expected to improve. Neither bloodletting nor cupping was an effective treatment for illness. Not surprisingly, many patients who underwent such treatments died anyway.

Herbal Treatments

Not all treatments were as painful as bloodletting and cupping. Medieval doctors also gave herbal tonics, or potions, to their patients. It was believed that every substance found in nature had a powerful and sometimes healing property. Doctors mixed tonics out of hundreds of substances, including such strange things as earthworms, dirt, and urine. Most of these tonics had little medical value, and some were dangerous or even deadly.

Religious Treatments

Other treatments for illness were of a religious nature. Many people believed that if they prayed to God, the punishment of illness would be lifted. Ill people would also take pilgrimages, or trips, to holy and healing lands in the hope that they would be cured.

Changing Views About Illness and Death

When the plague struck Europe, it became obvious that accepted medical treatments were not saving people from dying. Bloodletting, potions, prayers, and other traditional remedies were simply not effective in curing the plague. It also became clear that even if the plague was the result of God's wrath, it affected sinners and those without sin equally. People discovered that you could get the plague by being in the same room with a plague-infected person. As a result of this discovery, many people abandoned their friends and family members who were infected with the plague. People on newly docked ships were forced to stay on board the ship for a period of time until it was certain that the plague was not on the ship.

In addition to avoiding contact with people infected with the plague, people also performed more superstitious practices in order to stay healthy. One such practice was the wearing of costumes. People

Medieval doctors believed that costumes like the one pictured at left would protect them from the plague.

wrongly believed that certain costumes could protect them from becoming infected. Other protective devices, such as flea traps, were also commonly used as a way to avoid infection.

Before the occurrence of the Black Death, death was often viewed as the final part of life before joining God. Before the plague, literature and art often compared death to a kind friend or gentle being. After the plague years,

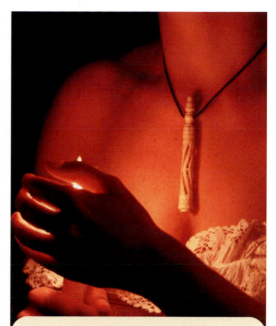

It was hoped that the blood-soaked cloth inside this ivory flea trap would attract plague-carrying fleas away from the wearer.

literature and art reflected the attitude that death was a painful and cruel enemy. Many paintings of the time show the character of death as a frightening and horrid figure.

1

THE BUBONIC PLAGUE: WHAT WE KNOW

The word "plague" comes from the Latin word *plaga*, which means "wound" or "pestilence." A pestilence is a deadly epidemic disease. The bubonic plague can be either an epidemic or a pandemic disease. An epidemic disease is a disease that affects a large number of people in a specific area at the same time. A pandemic disease is a disease that is spread over an entire country, continent, or even the whole world. The Black Death was a pandemic disease.

At the time of the Black Death, it was believed that there was a single, deadly plague. Many historians now believe that the Black Death was caused by more than one form of plague. When people suffer from the same illness, they will also suffer from similar symptoms. While the bubonic plague was the form that is most often described in the written accounts from people who lived during the Black Death, there are also written accounts of symptoms that are not characteristic of the bubonic form. These non-bubonic symptoms are believed to have been caused by other forms of plague.

The bubonic and other forms of plague have not disappeared from the earth. Plague still can and does develop, but today we know much more about it than did our ancestors. Advances in medicine and research have allowed us to learn that plagues, as well as other illnesses, have direct scientific causes. By knowing the direct cause of an illness, such as an insect bite, we can learn ways to avoid that illness. Discovering the cause also helps doctors and scientists to find a cure for the illness. Scientists continue to research illnesses in order to find direct causes. Scientists also look for ways of controlling the causes so that they don't infect or harm us too seriously.

What Causes the Bubonic Plague

The bubonic plague is caused by bacteria. Bacteria are microscopic organisms. Microscopic means that they are so small you can see them only by examining them under a microscope. A microbiologist studies microscopic organisms. The study of bacteria is a very important science because there are many different kinds of bacteria. Each kind of bacteria has its own unique effect on other living organisms.

At any time, there are millions of bacteria living around, on, and inside of us. Some types of bacteria are harmless, while other kinds can cause disease and even death. Some forms of harmless bacteria help the body to perform important functions, such as digesting food. Harmful bacteria, however, can cause sore throats, infections, and cavities in teeth. Harmful bacteria release poisons that cause a variety of symptoms, including the swollen lymph nodes of the bubonic plague.

Yersinia Pestis

The bacterium that causes the bubonic plague is called *Yersinia pestis*. This bacterium is named after Alexandre Yersin, the Swiss microbiologist who discovered it. In 1894 there was a violent outbreak of the bubonic plague in Hong Kong. Yersin, who was working in French Indochina at the time, hurried to Hong Kong and set up a temporary laboratory. He examined the bodies of people who had died of the plague. By studying tissue samples that he took from the buboes (swollen lymph glands) and organs of the deceased victims, he was able to locate the microorganism that caused the plague.

Yersin published his findings later that year. At the same time, another microbiologist, named Shibasaburo Kitasato, published his own findings on the bacteria. Many people feel that Yersin's research findings are more accurate than Kitasato's findings. For many years, the bacteria was called *Pasteurella bacilla* after the Pasteur Institute of Paris, where Yersin had been a student and lab assistant. Recently, *Yersinia pestis* has become an accepted name for the bacteria in the medical community.

Symptoms of the Plague

The bubonic plague causes buboes to form in the human body. A bubo is a swollen, darkened, and often painful lymph node. Lymph nodes—also called

Alexandre Yersin discovered the bacterium that causes the bubonic plague.

lymph glands—are located in various parts of our bodies. Some can be felt just beneath the skin, while others are found deep inside the body. Lymph nodes hold special cells that destroy and kill bacteria and

- ✪ The word "bacterium" is the singular form of the word "bacteria."
- ✪ A bacterium is a germ.
- ✪ Germs are microorganisms, some of which can cause illness.
- ✪ Types of germs include bacteria, viruses, protozoa, fungi, and parasites.
- ✪ Harmful bacteria can be killed by many antibiotic medicines.
- ✪ Harmless bacteria aid in returning needed elements to our atmosphere.
- ✪ Harmless bacteria decompose, or separate, waste and dead organisms.
- ✪ Some forms of bacteria can live off of a host but do nothing to harm or help the host.

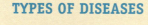

TYPES OF DISEASES

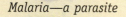

Malaria—a parasite

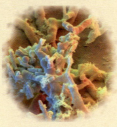

Athlete's Foot— a fungus

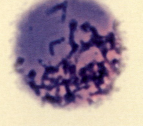

Polio—a virus

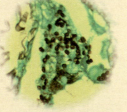

AIDS-related pneumonia—a protozoa

Cholera—a bacterium

viruses that get into the body. The bubonic plague causes an infected person's lymph nodes to swell, sometimes becoming as large as an egg or an apple. The most common area of swelling from the plague is in the groin area, which is how the bubonic plague was named—the Greek word for "groin" is *boubon*. Other noticeable swellings can occur in the lymph nodes of the armpits and on the back of the neck.

2

THE TRANSMISSION OF THE PLAGUE

Just like every other living organism on this planet, bacteria have the need to survive. In order for bacteria to survive, they need a place to live that will protect them and allow them to multiply. Bacteria also need sugars, vitamins, chemicals, and minerals in order to live. These nutrients can be found in the bodies of other living organisms such as plants, animals, and humans. To survive, a bacterium will find another living organism, or a host, from which it can obtain nutrition and a safe place to live. Some bacteria can also be found living in soil and water.

A struggle for life occurs when a bacterium enters a host. The cells and organs of a body work to protect the body from harmful things.

Some bacteria are allowed to survive in a host body because the body knows that those bacteria are harmless. Bacteria that are harmful or damaging to the host, however, are selected by the body to be killed. Most bacteria want to keep their host alive because the body is their source for nutrition. Harmful bacteria will cause infections, illness, and death despite the fact that they need to keep their host alive. Harmful bacteria produce and release poisons, or toxins, into the body, which can cause any number of symptoms.

In order to get into the body of a host, bacteria must come into contact with the host. Different kinds of bacteria can come into contact with a host in different ways.

Consuming Contaminated Food or Water

A host can be infected with bacteria by consuming contaminated food or water. Bacteria live in the contaminated food and water. When we eat contaminated food or drink contaminated water, we allow the bacteria into our bodies. Contaminated food and water help to transmit the bacteria into our bodies.

Through the Air in Dust or Liquid Droplets

Bacteria can also be transmitted to a host through dust and liquid droplets in the air. Liquid droplets can be found in your breath. A person infected with certain kinds of bacteria can transmit them to you through his or her breath by coughing or sneezing.

Direct Physical Contact

Bacteria can enter a host through direct contact. Bacteria can enter through scratches or openings in the skin. The bacteria can be on or in any person, animal, or item that the host handles or has direct physical contact with.

Through a Vector

Bacteria can enter the host by using a vector. A vector is another organism or insect that bites or scratches the surface of the skin of the host. When the skin is punctured, the wound can act as a doorway that lets the bacteria into the host. The vector might also deposit a fluid that contains the bacteria.

How the Plague Is Transmitted

It was not known in earlier centuries, but *Yersinia pestis* can be transmitted through a vector, direct physical contact, and liquid droplets. The plague is transmitted to humans from animals through a vector or direct physical contact. Once in the human population, the plague can be transmitted from person to person through liquid droplets.

The plague bacterium can be found in some wild animals. Wild animals carrying the bacteria are located in some areas of Asia, Africa, southeastern Europe, and North and South America. These wild animals can carry *Yersinia pestis* without getting sick or experiencing symptoms. Since wild animals carry the bacteria but do not get sick or die, it means that these animals have a resistance to the bacteria. Bears, coyotes, badgers, skunks, and raccoons are examples of wild animals that can carry the bacteria but are resistant to the sickness caused by the bacteria.

At some point, an infected wild animal may have contact with a rat or rodent population living in or near cities and towns. Plague epidemics occur when bacteria spread from infected wild animals to rat or rodent populations. The plague is transmitted from the wild animals to other animals through a vector or through direct physical contact. The rat or rodent populations are not as resistant to the bacteria as the wild animals. The bacteria can cause a plague among the rat or rodent population. Animals, such as cats and dogs that come into contact with infected rats and rodents, can also become infected.

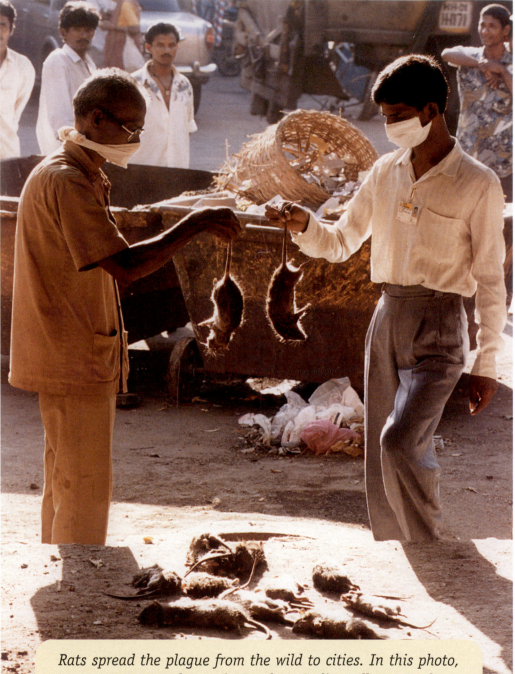

Rats spread the plague from the wild to cities. In this photo, government employees in Bombay, India, collect rats that will be dissected and checked for Yersinia pestis *bacteria during a 1994 plague outbreak.*

The Vector That Transmits the Plague

Yersinia pestis is most commonly transmitted through a vector. The flea is the vector for the plague. Fleas drink the blood of other organisms in order to survive. Fleas transmit the plague after biting an infected rat or other infected animal. There are several different species, or varieties, of fleas. About 100 flea varieties are known to be carriers of *Yersinia pestis*. Not all of the carrying varieties can pass the bacteria along, or act as vectors of the plague. There are thirty-one varieties of fleas that have been proven to be vectors of the plague.

When a flea bites an animal, it draws blood into its body for a meal. When a flea bites a plague-infected rat or animal, the plague bacteria also enter the flea's body. The bacteria multiply and grow so quickly that the flea's gut becomes clogged. When the flea's gut is clogged, the flea is not able to digest the blood. When the flea bites a new host, it tries to draw blood in but ends up releasing the blood that it could not digest into the new host. The blood that goes into the new host will carry the *Yersinia pestis* bacteria with it, which in turn infect the new host with the plague.

As the rat or rodent populations die out, the fleas must search for new food sources. Since rat and rodent populations live near humans, humans are often the

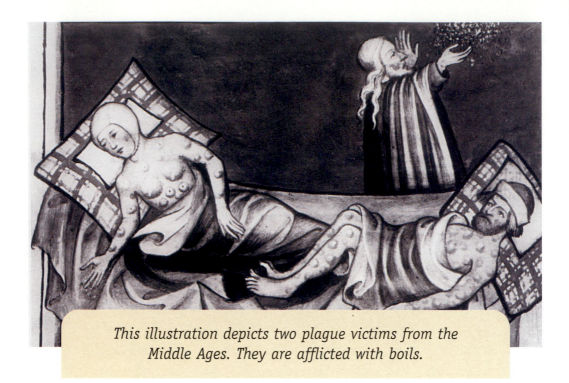

This illustration depicts two plague victims from the Middle Ages. They are afflicted with boils.

next source of nutrients for the infected fleas. When the flea finds its human host, it bites through the skin to draw blood. The infected blood that the flea was not able to digest will be released into the human host. The blood carries *Yersinia pestis* through the bite wound and into the new human host.

The Bubonic Bacteria in Human Hosts

The bite area where the bacteria enter the human host will swell and become infected. The bacteria kill healthy cells near the wound, which causes a

1894

The organism that causes the bubonic plague is discovered by Alexandre Yersin. Yersin also discovers the fact that rats are affected by plague shortly before the plague strikes humans. The organism is also discovered by Japanese microbiologist Shibasaburo Kitasato.

1897

The Japanese physician Masanori Ogata suggests that fleas could be possible vectors for the plague.

Later that year, P. L. Simond proves that fleas are the vectors for the plague. Simond observes small bites on the legs of plague victims, and demonstrates that the bites bring about the bubonic swelling. Simond conducts an experiment in which a healthy rat is brought into contact with a rat that has been killed by the plague. Simond discovers that the healthy rat becomes infected when fleas jump from the dead rat to the healthy rat.

1896

The first plague vaccine is made by the Russian scientist Waldemar Haffkine.

darkened blister to form. *Yersinia pestis* spreads from the blister to the nearest lymph nodes. In most cases, the bacteria grow faster than the body can fight them. The lymph nodes become hot, sore, dark in color, and swollen as infection sets in. Within hours of infection the bacteria spread into the bloodstream, which allows the bacteria to be delivered throughout the body. The infected person may also experience high fever, delirium, headaches, and hemorrhages. Hemorrhages are discharges of blood under the skin, usually dark purple or black in color. Darkened skin on the hands and feet may also develop. Some historical sources believe that the term Black Death came from the fact that the skin and buboes turn dark colors.

If the infection is left untreated, bacteria can invade the lungs, which causes the pneumonic form of the plague. Pneumonia is an infection of the lungs. The pneumonic form of the bubonic plague is a very serious and rapidly fatal illness. A *Yersinia pestis* infection of the lungs causes difficulty in breathing, severe coughing, and vomiting of blood. During the coughing fits, the infected person releases large amounts of the *Yersinia pestis* into the air. *Yersinia pestis* can also be released into the air when an infected person sneezes. When *Yersinia pestis* is transmitted through liquid droplets or the air, the bacteria enter directly into the

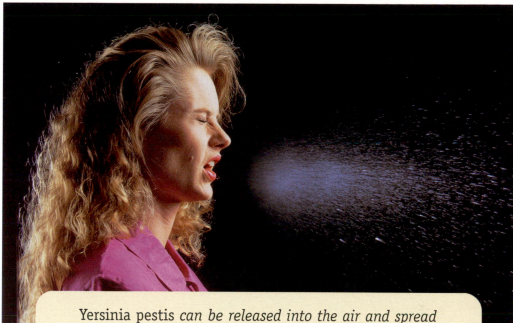

Yersinia pestis can be released into the air and spread when an infected person sneezes.

lungs of the new host. The new host's lungs become infected with *Yersinia pestis*. When the bacteria infect the lungs first, the pneumonic form of the plague develops rather than the bubonic form.

Yersinia pestis can also enter into the bloodstream in such large amounts that it can cause another form of the plague called septicemia. The bacteria invade and overpower the bloodstream. A rash will appear on the skin, and the host may die before any symptoms of the bubonic plague, such as swollen buboes, can appear. The septicemic form of the plague kills a host very quickly because the bacteria are literally taking over the body.

THE HISTORY OF THE PLAGUE

Written accounts of illnesses and plagues ravaging cities, countries, and continents can be found throughout history. Perhaps the earliest written account of the plague is found in the First Book of Samuel in the Bible. Historians study writings about plagues in order to determine the type of plague that struck and where it struck. Depending on how detailed the written information is, historians may be able to piece together a plague history.

AD 541—The Great Pandemic, or Justinian's Plague

Historians believe that the first worldwide, or pandemic, plague occurred during the sixth century.

During this time, the Byzantine Empire was ruled by Justinian, which is why this plague is often called Justinian's plague. Much of our knowledge about this plague is taken from the writings of a legal advisor named Procopius. Procopius was traveling on a series of missions throughout the Mediterranean during the time of the pandemic outbreak.

Procopius wrote that the plague started in Pelusium, which was an Egyptian city at the easternmost mouth of the Nile River. The plague then swept westward across Mediterranean Europe. People from Constantinople to Spain were ravaged. Procopius observed that all of the victims of the plague suffered the

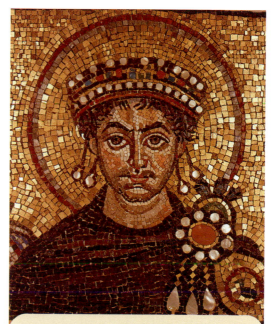

The first pandemic plague occurred in the sixth century, during the reign of the Byzantine emperor Justinian.

same symptoms. His writings mention the bubo swellings in the armpits, groin, and neck areas.

In Constantinople, the capital of the Byzantine Empire, the bodies of plague victims were so numerous that disposing of them became a problem in itself. Some were burned, while others were buried in mass graves or thrown into bodies of water. In many areas the number of corpses became so great that many were simply placed on rooftops while others were left to rot in their homes.

Historians now believe that Justinian's plague originated in central Africa, rather than in Pelusium itself. The epidemic is believed to have been carried northward, through Pelusium and into Europe. Even after the pandemic plague ceased, occasional plague outbreaks occurred throughout the Mediterranean region during the rest of the sixth century.

The Fourteenth Century— The Black Death

Historians believe that the Black Death started in Asia and then spread westward into Europe. An epidemic of the plague originated in northeastern China in 1334. This plague eventually killed two-thirds of China's inhabitants. The plague then spread west across China, through the Middle East, and into the countries along the eastern Mediterranean. The plague spread along the trade routes, such as the Silk Road from China and the Rhine trade routes of Europe. The plague spread freely by ship and by

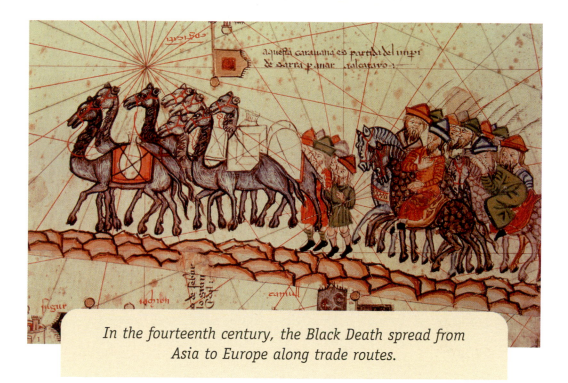

In the fourteenth century, the Black Death spread from Asia to Europe along trade routes.

land, wherever there was a source of people or rats to carry the disease.

The plague first reached Europe, or more specifically the Italian peninsula, in 1347. The plague was brought to Italy by merchant ships that had returned from Kaffa, a Genoese trading port on the Black Sea. An army that wished to drive the Genoese out of Kaffa had been attacking the port.

When the attacking army developed the plague, they catapulted the infected corpses of their soldiers over the walls and into Kaffa. The Genoese dumped the infected bodies into the water as quickly as possible, but it was too late. The plague set in at Kaffa, infecting the people who lived there.

The Catholic Church believes in honoring people who have lived their lives in order to serve God. The church honors some of these people by giving them the title of Saint. The tradition of sainthood dates back to AD 100. This practice came from the early Jewish tradition of honoring prophets and holy people with shrines. The first Christian saints were martyrs, or people who were persecuted and killed because of their Christian beliefs.

There are several saints who were chosen to represent the plague and plague epidemics. Some of these saints had personal experiences with the plague while they were living. Macarius of Antioch died of the plague. Saint Roch tended to people with the plague. He also became infected with the plague, but did not die from it. Aloysius Gonzaga tended to plague victims in Rome and later died of the plague. The following is a list of the plague saints and the calendar days on which they are celebrated. Some saints are known by more than one name. Other names are given in parenthesis.

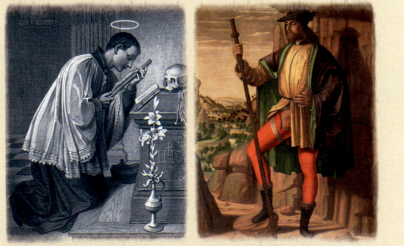

Aloysius Gonzaga   Saint Roch

SAINT	CALENDAR DAY
Catald (Cathal)	May 10
Cuthbert	March 20
Edmund of East Anglia	November 20
Francis of Paola	April 2
Francis Xavier	December 3
George (Victory Bringer)	April 23
Godebertha (Godeberta of Noyon, Godberta)	April 11
Aloysius Gonzaga (Luigi Gonzaga)	June 21
Gregory the Great (Gregory I, Father of Fathers)	September 3
Macarius of Antioch (Macaire of Ghent)	April 10
Roch (Rock, Rocco, Roque, Rochus, Rollox)	August 16
Sebastian	January 20
Valentine of Rome (Valentine of Terni)	February 14
Walburga* (Bugga, Gaudurge, Walpurgis)	February 25

* Walburga is also celebrated on May 1, September 24, and October 12.

Hoping to escape the plague that was spreading throughout Kaffa, four Genoese ships returned to the Italian peninsula. Tragically, the four ships were contaminated with the plague. When the ships docked, the plague was spread to Italy.

From its foothold on the Italian peninsula, the plague quickly spread northward into central Europe. By 1348 the populations of Paris, England, Ireland, and Germany were being ravaged by the disease. The plague was carried further north into Norway and Scotland in 1349 and east into Russia two years later. By 1352, the plague had almost formed a complete circle around Europe, reaching the Russian city of Kiev, which was located just 700 kilometers north of Kaffa. For the next four centuries, the plague reappeared

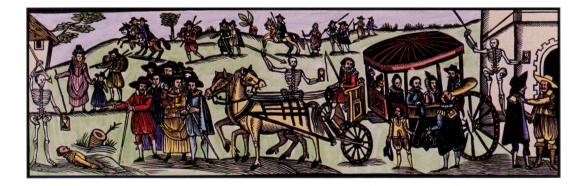

This 1630 engraving shows townspeople attempting to flee and escape the plague.

in smaller outbreaks throughout Eurasia (Europe and Asia) every twenty years or so.

The Black Death Spreads Hatred

The cause of the Black Death was not known during the time it was devastating the towns and cities of fourteenth-century Europe. This ignorance filled people with fear and led to wild and false beliefs about the cause of the plague. Many people absurdly came to believe that the plague had been started by the Jews. It was believed that Jews deliberately created the plague because they wanted to destroy Christians. This belief grew out of centuries of prejudice against Jews.

When the plague struck, the general public started to blame Jews for the disease. Jews were accused of poisoning the water, which was believed to have caused the sickness. This accusation led to the persecution and murder of many innocent Jews. Many Jews were taken captive and tortured until they agreed that they had poisoned the water.

Some Christians did not believe that the Jews had poisoned the water but rather that the plague was a punishment sent directly from God. Many Christians believed that God was angry with them for tolerating the Jews. A group of people called the flagellants believed that they could lift the punishment. The flagellants traveled from village to village, parading in

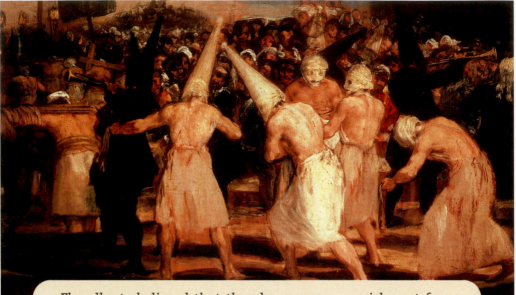

Flagellants believed that the plague was a punishment from God for tolerating the Jews. They traveled from town to town, whipping themselves as a form of penance and persecuting Jews.

the streets while whipping themselves. They whipped themselves to show God their sorrow for tolerating the Jews. In each town, flagellants furthered the blame of the Jews. In many cases, the flagellants would run the Jews out of town or even murder them. Some flagellants would even attack non-Jews who tried to protect Jews from harm.

Not all Christians blamed the Jews for the plague. Pope Clement VI announced that the flagellants were wrong in their slaughter of the Jews. He pointed out the fact that Jews were dying of the plague in the same way that Christians were. Clement VI called for the arrest of all flagellants. King Philip VI also showed his dislike of the flagellants by passing a regulation forbidding public flagellation on penalty of death. The flagellants fled to avoid arrest and death, but the flagellant practice never completely disappeared and would crop up from time to time during other occurrences of the plague over the next century.

During the course of the plague, thousands of Jews were exiled from or murdered in Germany, Belgium, Holland, and other parts of Europe. In Strasbourg, more than two thousand Jews were asked to convert to Christianity. Those who refused were tied to stakes and burned to death. Small children were pulled from the fire and baptized as the parents died. In some villages, Jews set their own houses on fire and killed themselves.

1893—The Modern Pandemic

The third great pandemic started in the south of China in 1893. This outbreak of the plague was spread by caravan and river routes to the great Chinese cities of Hong Kong and Canton. By 1896, it had spread west into the cities of Singapore and Bombay. The plague was also carried south into the Malay Peninsula and the Philippine Islands. Far-reaching trade routes carried the plague from southern Asia to Europe, Africa, North and South America, and

THE POPULAR CHILDREN'S RHYME
Ring around the Rosies,
A pocket full of Posies,
Achoo! Achoo!
We all fall down.

This popular children's rhyme grew out of medieval beliefs about the plague. The first line refers to the rash that occurred when a person had the plague. The second line is about posies, which people would carry in the pockets of their clothes during the plague. It was believed that the smell of these flowers could cover up the corrupt vapors thought to have caused the plague. The last two lines describe the sickness and eventual death brought about by the plague.

THE BARBER SHOP POLE
The origin of the pole outside of many barber shops dates back to the time of medieval bloodletting. The red and white stripes are symbolic of the process of bloodletting, which was often performed by barbers in the Middle Ages. Bloodletting was a popular medieval medical treatment. It was done in an effort to cure illnesses such as the Black Plague. The red stripe symbolizes blood, while the white stripe symbolizes the piece of cloth that was tied around the cut limb in order to stop the blood flow. The pole itself is shaped like the rod that a bloodletting patient squeezed. Squeezing the rod increased the flow of blood to the cut.

Australia. By 1900, cities as far from China as Buenos Aires, Rio de Janeiro, and San Francisco experienced outbreaks of the plague.

It's estimated that 20 million people died over the course of the next seventy-five years from the pandemic and from occasional plague outbreaks that followed. It was during this outbreak of the plague that Alexandre Yersin and Shibasaburo Kitasato discovered the organism that causes the disease. At the time, it wasn't known that fleas can transmit the plague from infected rats to humans. However, a physician named Mary Miles observed that rats in China were struck

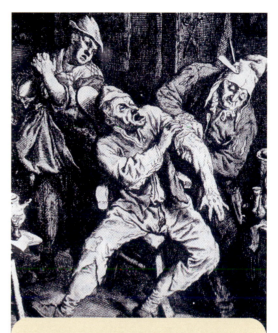

Bloodletting was performed by barbers during the Middle Ages.

with the plague as well as humans. It was also noted that rats came out of their holes in broad daylight, stumbled about as if in a daze, and then died.

Occurrence of the Plague Today

The plague still occurs occasionally throughout the world. Individual cases of bubonic plague, about fifteen a year, are reported in the western parts of the United States. These cases occur in parts of New Mexico, Arizona, Colorado, California, Oregon, and Nevada. These cases of infection are the result of people coming into contact with plague-infected wild animals or rodents. The last plague outbreak happened in Los Angeles in 1924.

Plague infection also occurs in Africa, South America, and Asia. The World Health Organization reports that there are 1,000 to 3,000 cases of plague throughout the world each year. Because the plague still exists today, certain measures have been taken to ensure that widespread epidemics do not occur. The International Health Agreement, which is an agreement between the countries of the world, requires all health authorities to report new cases of the plague within twenty-four hours. Immediate reporting of plague cases throughout the world ensures that measures can be taken to prevent the plague from spreading.

PLAGUE DIAGNOSIS AND TREATMENT

We know a lot more about the plague today than people of the medieval age did. Research has allowed us to learn what causes the plague. We now know how to diagnose, treat, and even prevent the plague. We have also learned about the conditions that put us at an increased risk for another plague epidemic.

Who Can Get the Plague?

Anybody who has had exposure to plague-infected wild animals can contract the disease. People and animals that come into contact with, or even get near, rodents that have died from the plague are at risk for getting the disease. When an animal dies of the plague, the disease

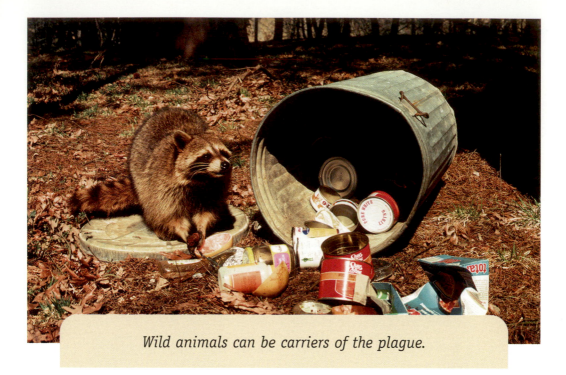

Wild animals can be carriers of the plague.

is carried on by the infected fleas that lived on the animal. The fleas, searching for a host body, will jump onto any animal or human that happens to get close enough. A person can also get the plague if he or she has scratches, or other skin openings, and comes into direct contact with a plague-infected animal or person. House pets can also bring the plague or plague infested fleas into the home. A person can become infected either through indirect or direct physical contact with an infected house pet.

Diagnosis

Plague infections require an immediate diagnosis, as death from the plague can take place in as little as three days from the time of infection. A doctor attempting to diagnose the disease will look for these classic symptoms:

- A general feeling of sickness
- High fever
- Chills
- Headaches
- Delirium
- Helplessness
- Hemorrhages under the skin
- Darkened skin on the hands and legs
- Painful or tender swollen lymph nodes
- White coating on the tongue
- Marked sensitivity to light

If a doctor feels that a patient may have the plague, the doctor is required by law to isolate the patient from everyone else. The patient will be hospitalized and undergo laboratory tests. There are different tests for the different forms of the plague. The doctor will have samples of the patient's blood, lymph glands, or saliva examined for presence of the plague bacteria.

If the results show that the patient has the plague, certain steps are taken to keep it from spreading. People who have been in close contact with the patient will be identified and evaluated for the possibility of infection. All suspected and actual cases of the plague are reported to local and state health departments. Diagnosis of the plague is usually confirmed by the Centers for Disease Control and Prevention (CDC). The CDC reports all U.S. plague cases to the World Health Organization.

Treatment

Immediate treatment for the plague is very important in order to ensure the patient's survival. As soon as the plague is suspected, doctors will prescribe an antibiotic for the patient. An antibiotic is a medication that does not allow bacteria to survive and multiply in an infected person.

Some antibiotics can also be given before the disease is contracted, as a preventative measure. These antibiotics are called prophylactic antibiotics. The word "prophylactic" means protection. Prophylactic antibiotics can keep people from developing the plague if they become exposed to it in the near future. These antibiotics are given to people to protect them from getting the plague, rather than to treat them for plague infection. Prophylactic antibiotics might also be given to anyone who has had, or will have, close exposure to an infected patient. Doctors will also give prophylactic antibiotics to anyone who will be traveling to an area of the world where a plague outbreak is occurring. This will ensure that the person does not become infected with the plague even though he or she is exposed to it.

Vaccines for the plague are available, but they are used in limited amounts. In order for a person to be vaccinated against the plague, they need to receive multiple shots over a period of many months. Because vaccines take time to work, they cannot be used for immediate protection against the plague. Vaccines are more effective for people who need long-term protection from the plague because they are exposed to it on a regular basis. Scientists who handle and study *Yersinia pestis* and people who handle infected animals as part of their work are among those people who are commonly vaccinated against the plague.

PREVENTION OF THE PLAGUE

The plague is a controllable and avoidable disease among human populations. Exposure to the plague from a rodent or wild animal population is also controllable. If the plague is present in an environment, there are precautions that can be taken to ensure that the plague does not develop into an epidemic or pandemic disease.

Outbreaks commonly occur in areas of the world where housing and sanitation conditions are poor. The word "sanitation" means the protection of good health by keeping living conditions clean. Rats and rodents often live in areas where sanitation conditions are poor, and contact with plague-infected rodents is very dangerous to humans.

Environmental Sanitation

The very first step that we can take in reducing the risk of being exposed to the plague is to control the number of rodents and fleas in and near the areas where we live. Keeping good sanitation conditions will ensure that rodents are not drawn to these areas. This is called environmental sanitation. The first step of environmental sanitation is to protect food sources that could attract rats and rodents. By making garbage and pet food sources tamperproof, we can reduce the number of rodents that will be drawn to these food sources.

The second step of environmental sanitation is to remove all junk piles from areas where people live. These junk piles offer rodents a place to build their nests. By removing the piles, we can make it harder for rodents to find shelter.

There are various poisons that can also be used to keep rodent populations under control. These powerful chemicals should be used only by professionals as they are harmful to humans as well. Using disinfectants and cleaning agents in and around our homes on a regular basis is another way to keep good sanitation conditions.

Public Awareness and Action

Although it has been attempted, killing wild animals that may be carriers of the plague is costly and very difficult to do. People who live in areas near wild animal populations that are known to carry the plague should be aware of how to avoid exposure. These people should also keep an eye out for plague activity in local rodent populations. A sure sign of plague activity among rodent populations is a large number of rodent deaths. It is important that people report any cases of sick or dead animals to their local health department or law enforcement agency. Trained professionals who know how to handle the possibility of disease will investigate the animal deaths.

Other actions that people can take to ensure that they don't contract the plague are:

- Treating pets with flea control on a regular basis, either through flea collars or flea powders. Pets should also be regularly inspected for fleas.

- Limiting the number of times that pets are allowed to freely roam outdoors.

- Telling authorities immediately if contact is made with a possibly plague-infected animal. If for any reason the animal has to be handled, gloves should always be worn on the hands of the person handling the animal.

- Wearing flea repellent on skin and clothing when traveling to areas where exposure to the plague is possible.

- Removing junk piles and potential food sources around the home that could attract rodents.

- Wearing gloves and using a strong disinfectant or cleaner while cleaning areas that wild animals have infested. The entire area should be wet with cleaner. Any remains or animal materials should be disposed of in sealed bags.

Traveling Precautions

People who travel to areas where animals or humans are known to have the plague should take precautions to lower their risk of becoming infected. Travelers can take prophylactic antibiotics before their trips to strengthen their resistance to the plague. Travelers should avoid any areas where recent human cases have occurred. People should also avoid areas where dead rats have been found and avoid handling any sick or dead animals from those areas. Bug repellents should be applied to clothing, skin, and bedding accommodations.

GLOSSARY

antibiotic   Medicine that destroys the growth
   of bacteria.
bacteria   Microorganisms that can be harmful or
   harmless to other living things.
Black Death   The bubonic plague.
bloodletting   Bleeding for a medical purpose.
bubo   A swelling in the lymph glands of the neck,
   armpit, or groin.
consumption   The act of eating or drinking.
contagious   Can be spread through contact.
epidemic   The sudden breaking out of a disease in
   a particular area, affecting many people at the
   same time.
flagellant   A person who whips himself or herself
   for religious purposes.

hemorrhage   A discharge or release of blood.

humor   Any of the four body fluids believed by the Romans and Greeks to influence health and personality.

infectious   Something or someone contaminated with disease that can spread to other organisms.

lymph nodes   Infection fighting centers of the body, also known as lymph glands.

medieval   Of the middle ages.

microbiologist   A scientist who studies microorganisms.

microorganism   A very small organism, or living thing.

pandemic   Universal or global; worldwide.

peninsula   A piece of land almost surrounded by water.

persecution   Mistreatment because of religious beliefs or race.

plague   Any of a variety of strong, deadly, and contagious diseases.

pneumonic plague   A form of plague that infects the lungs.

prophylactic antibiotic   Any antibiotic that is used to prevent the plague, rather than to treat the plague.

quarantine   To forcibly isolate someone or restrict someone's contact with others.

resistance   An ability to resist something such as a disease.

sanitation   Keeping surroundings clean to maintain good health.

septicemia   A form of the plague that infects the bloodstream.

species   Varieties of an animal or plant.

tonic   A medicine meant to restore good heath.

trade route   A route, by sea or land, used by traders.

transmission   To pass from one source to another.

vapor   A cloudy substance in the air.

vector   A transmitter of microorganisms from one animal or species to another.

wrath   Extreme rage or violence accompanied by an intent to punish.

FOR MORE INFORMATION

In the United States

Centers for Disease Control and Prevention (CDC)
1600 Clifton Rd.
Atlanta, GA 30333
Public inquiries by phone:
(404) 639-3534
(800) 311-3435
Web site: http://www.cdc.gov

The CDC is an agency of the Department of Health and Human Services. The mission of the CDC is to promote health and quality of life by controlling and preventing disease, injury, and disability. The CDC Web site includes information about the plague, its history, risk, prevention, treatment, and diagnosis, as well as information on many other diseases.

Division of Vector-Borne Infectious Diseases (DVBID),
and the National Center for Infectious Diseases (NCID)
P.O. Box 2087
Fort Collins, CO 80522
Public Inquiries: (800) 311-3435, (404) 639-3534
E-mail for the DVBID: dvbid@cdc.gov
E-mail for the NCID: ncid@cdc.gov

The DVBID is a division of the NCID, which is part of
the CDC, or Centers for Disease Control and Prevention. The mission of the NCID is to prevent illness,
disability, and death caused by infectious diseases in
the United States and the world. The DVBID and NCID
Web sites are part of the CDC web site and can be
accessed through http://www.cdc.gov.

In Canada

Health Canada
Tunney's Pasture
A.L. 0904A
Ottowa, ON K1A 0K9
(613) 957-2991
E-mail: info@www.hc-sc.gc.ca
Web site: http://www.hc-sc.gc.ca
Health Canada promotes disease prevention and
enhances healthy living for all Canadians. Health

Canada also enforces health laws and ensures that health care services are available to every Canadian. The Health Canada Web site includes information on the plague and other diseases and illnesses.

Bureau of Infectious Diseases, Laboratory Centre for
      Disease Control
Health Protection Branch
Health Canada
Tunney's Pasture
Ottowa, ON K1A 0L2
Postal Locator: 0603E1
Web site: http://www.hc-sc.gc.ca/hpb/lcdc/bid/index.html

The Bureau of Infectious Diseases is a division of the Laboratory Centre for Disease Control, which is a part of Health Canada. The bureau researches and checks for infectious diseases. The bureau works to identify, prevent, and control infectious diseases throughout Canada.

FOR FURTHER READING

Giblin, James. *When Plague Strikes: The Black Death, Smallpox, AIDS*. New York: HarperCollins Children's Books, 1995.

Lamond, Margrete. *Plague and Pestilence: Deadly Diseases That Changed the World (True Stories)*. Saint Leonards, Australia: Allen & Unwin, 1997.

McDonald, Fiona. *How Would You Survive in the Middle Ages?* Danbury, CT: Franklin Watts, Inc., 1997.

Roden, Katie, Richard Rockwood, and Rob Shone. *The Plague*. Bridgeport, CT: Copper Beech Books, 1996.

INDEX

CREDITS

About the Author

Holly Cefrey is a New York-based freelance writer who has authored a number of books on medical and health related topics.

Photo Credits

Cover © LeBeau/Custom Medical Stock Photo; p. 4 © Museo del Prado, Madrid, Spain/Giraudon, Paris/Superstock; pp. 12, 42, and 46 © SuperStock; p. 14 © EpConcepts/Custom Medical Stock Photo; p. 15 © Nicole Duplaix/Corbis; p. 19 © Leonard de Selva/Corbis; p. 20 top left and bottom right © Custom Medical Stock Photo, bottom left © Dr. M Klein/Peter Arnold, Inc., top right © CNRI/Science Photo Library/Photo Researchers, middle © David Scharf/Peter Arnold, Inc; p. 26 © Associated Press;

p. 28 © Bettmann/Corbis; p. 29 © Corbis Royalty Free; p. 31 © Matt Meadows/ Peter Arnold, Inc. p. 33 © Musee de Chartres, France/Explorer, Paris/Super-Stock; p. 35 © Bibliotheque Nationale, Paris, France/ET Archive, London/SuperStock; p. 36 left © North Wind Picture Archives; p. 36 right © Arte & Immagini srl/Corbis; p. 38 © North Wind Picture Archives; p. 40 © Academia de San Fernando, Madrid, Spain/A.K.G., Berlin/SuperStock; p. 43 © J. Fishkin/Custom Medical Stock Photo.

Design and Layout

Evelyn Horovicz